Sensory Processing Disorder

Ashu Kumawat

Table of contents:

Understanding Sensory Processing Disorder

Sensory processing disorder (SPD), also known as sensory integration disorder, is a condition that affects how the brain processes and responds to sensory information from the environment. The sensory information includes sounds, sights, tastes, smells, textures, and movements. People with SPD may have difficulty organizing and interpreting sensory information, which can lead to challenges with behaviour, attention, and learning.

There are three types of sensory processing disorder: sensory modulation disorder, sensory discrimination disorder, and sensory-based motor disorder. Sensory modulation disorder refers to difficulties regulating the intensity, frequency, and duration of responses to sensory stimuli. Sensory discrimination disorder refers to challenges distinguishing between different sensory stimuli, such as sounds or textures. Sensory-based motor disorder refers to difficulties with coordination and planning of movement in response to sensory stimuli.

SPD can occur on its own, but it is also commonly associated with other neurodevelopmental disorders, such as autism spectrum disorder, attention-deficit/hyperactivity disorder (ADHD), and developmental coordination disorder.

Symptoms of SPD can vary widely depending on the individual and the type of sensory processing disorder they experience. Some common symptoms of SPD include:

Hypersensitivity to sensory input, such as loud noises or bright lights

Hyposensitivity to sensory input, such as not noticing when they are touched or not responding to pain

Difficulty processing sensory information, leading to sensory overload or shutdown

Difficulty with fine or gross motor coordination

Behavioural issues, such as tantrums, avoidance, or aggression

Challenges with attention and concentration

Delayed development of social and communication skills

Anxiety or depression related to sensory experiences

Understanding the symptoms of SPD is the first step in recognizing the condition and seeking appropriate treatment.

The exact causes of SPD are not yet fully understood, but research suggests that there may be genetic, environmental, and neurological factors involved. Some studies have identified specific genes that may be associated with sensory processing disorder, while other research has found links between prenatal and perinatal factors, such as premature birth or maternal stress, and an increased risk of SPD.

Neurologically, SPD is thought to be related to the way that the brain processes sensory information. Some studies have suggested that there may be differences in the way that the brains of people with SPD respond to sensory input, such as reduced activity in certain areas of the brain.

Diagnosing SPD can be challenging, as there is no specific test or set of criteria to identify the condition. Diagnosis usually involves a comprehensive assessment of the individual's sensory processing abilities, conducted by a trained professional such as an occupational therapist or a psychologist.

Treatment for SPD typically involves a combination of sensory integration therapy, occupational therapy, and behavioural therapy. Sensory integration therapy involves exposing the individual to different types of sensory stimuli in a controlled environment, with the goal of improving their ability to process and respond to sensory information. Occupational therapy can help individuals with SPD develop skills to manage daily activities, such as dressing and eating, that may be challenging due to sensory processing difficulties. Behavioural therapy can help individuals with SPD learn coping strategies and develop social skills.

In addition to these therapies, there are many strategies that individuals with SPD and their families can use to manage the challenges associated with the condition. These strategies may include creating a sensory-friendly environment at home and at school, using weighted blankets or compression clothing to provide calming sensory input, and developing routines to help reduce anxiety and provide predictability.

Living with sensory processing disorder can be challenging, but with the right treatment and support, individuals with SPD can learn to manage their symptoms and lead fulfilling lives. It is important for individuals with SPD and their families to seek out resources and support, and to advocate for their needs in school, work, and other settings.

The Role of Sensory Integration in Development

Sensory integration plays a crucial role in the development of the human brain and body. From birth, we are constantly receiving sensory input from our environment, which helps us to learn about the world around us and develop important skills such as coordination, balance, and communication.

Sensory integration refers to the process by which the brain receives, processes, and responds to sensory information from the environment. This information can come from a variety of sources, including vision, hearing, touch, taste, smell, and movement. Sensory integration allows the brain to organize and interpret this information, and to respond in a coordinated and appropriate way.

During early development, sensory integration is especially important for the formation of neural connections in the brain. In the first few years of life, the brain is rapidly developing and adapting to the environment, and sensory experiences play a critical role in this process. Babies and young children rely on sensory input to develop a range of skills, from motor coordination and balance to language and social interaction.

Sensory integration is closely linked to motor development, as sensory input helps to guide and refine motor movements. For example, the sense of touch helps babies to learn about the texture and shape of objects, which in turn helps them to develop the fine motor skills needed for grasping and manipulating objects. The sense of balance, or vestibular sense, helps children to develop their sense of spatial awareness and coordination, which is important for activities such as running, jumping, and climbing.

Sensory integration also plays a key role in the development of communication and social skills. From a young age, babies rely on social cues such as facial expressions and tone of voice to understand and communicate with others. These social cues are processed through the sensory system and help to develop important neural pathways related to social interaction and communication.

In addition to its role in early development, sensory integration continues to be important throughout the lifespan. As we grow and mature, our sensory experiences become more complex and varied, and our brains continue to adapt and learn from this input. Sensory integration can play a role in a wide range of activities and skills, from sports and exercise to artistic expression and problem-solving.

However, for individuals with sensory processing disorder (SPD), sensory integration can be challenging. SPD is a condition in which the brain has difficulty processing and responding to sensory information from the environment. This can lead to difficulties with motor coordination, communication, and social interaction, as well as challenges with behaviour and attention.

For individuals with SPD, sensory integration therapy can be an effective treatment option. Sensory integration therapy involves exposing the individual to a range of sensory experiences in a controlled and structured environment, with the goal of improving their ability to process and respond to sensory input. This therapy can help individuals with SPD to develop skills such as motor coordination, balance, and communication, and to manage the challenges associated with the condition.

In addition to therapy, there are many strategies that individuals with SPD and their families can use to support sensory integration. These may include creating a sensory-friendly environment at home and at school, providing opportunities for sensory play and exploration, and using sensory tools such as weighted blankets or compression clothing to provide calming input.

Overall, sensory integration plays a critical role in human development, from the earliest stages of life through adulthood. For individuals with sensory processing disorder, understanding and supporting sensory integration can be key to managing the challenges associated with the condition and achieving their full potential. With the right resources and support, individuals with SPD can develop the skills and abilities needed to thrive in a sensory-rich world.

Symptoms and Signs of Sensory Processing Disorder

Sensory Processing Disorder (SPD) is a condition in which the brain has difficulty processing and responding to sensory information from the environment. This can lead to a wide range of symptoms and signs that can impact daily life and overall functioning. In this chapter, we will explore the various symptoms and signs of SPD and how they may manifest in different individuals.

One of the primary symptoms of SPD is difficulty with sensory processing. This can manifest in a variety of ways, including hypersensitivity (overresponsiveness) or hyposensitivity (underresponsiveness) to sensory input. Hypersensitivity can lead to feelings of discomfort or even pain in response to stimuli such as bright lights, loud noises, or certain textures. Hyposensitivity can lead to a lack of awareness or response to sensory input, such as not feeling pain or temperature changes.

Another common symptom of SPD is difficulty with motor coordination and balance. This can manifest as clumsiness, poor spatial awareness, or difficulty with activities that require precise movements such as writing or using utensils. Individuals with SPD may also struggle with activities that involve movement or changes in position, such as riding in a car or swinging on a playground swing.

Communication and social difficulties are also common signs of SPD. For example, individuals with SPD may have difficulty with social interaction and may struggle to understand social cues such as facial expressions and tone of voice. They may also have difficulty with language development, including understanding and expressing language.

Behavioural difficulties are also common among individuals with SPD. These may include tantrums or meltdowns in response to sensory input, as well as difficulty with attention and concentration. Individuals with SPD may also exhibit repetitive behaviours or engage in self-stimulatory behaviour (such as rocking or spinning) as a way to manage sensory input.

In addition to these primary symptoms, there are a variety of secondary symptoms that can also be associated with SPD. These may include anxiety, depression, and sleep disturbances. Individuals with SPD may also struggle with academic and occupational performance, as well as overall quality of life.

It is important to note that the symptoms of SPD can vary widely among individuals, and not all individuals with SPD will experience the same set of symptoms or to the same degree. Additionally, SPD can often be mistaken for other conditions, such as autism spectrum disorder or attention deficit hyperactivity disorder (ADHD). For this reason, it is important to seek a professional evaluation from a qualified healthcare provider in order to receive an accurate diagnosis.

Despite the challenges associated with SPD, there are many treatment options available that can help individuals to manage their symptoms and improve their overall functioning. Sensory integration therapy, occupational therapy, and behavioural therapy are all commonly used to address the various symptoms and signs of SPD. Additionally, there are many strategies that individuals with SPD and their families can use to create a sensory-friendly environment at home and at school, such as providing opportunities for sensory play and exploration, using sensory tools such as weighted blankets or compression clothing, and avoiding or minimizing triggers for sensory overload.

In conclusion, sensory processing disorder is a complex condition that can impact individuals in a variety of ways. Understanding the various symptoms and signs of SPD is important in order to receive an accurate diagnosis and to identify effective treatment options. With the right resources and support, individuals with SPD can learn to manage their symptoms and thrive in a sensory-rich world.

Types of Sensory Processing Disorder

Sensory Processing Disorder (SPD) is a condition in which the brain has difficulty processing and responding to sensory information from the environment. There are three main types of SPD: Sensory Modulation Disorder, Sensory Discrimination Disorder, and Sensory-Based Motor Disorder. Each type of SPD is characterized by a specific set of symptoms and signs, and requires a unique approach to diagnosis and treatment.

Sensory Modulation Disorder

Sensory Modulation Disorder is the most common type of SPD, and it is characterized by difficulty with sensory processing regulation. This means that individuals with this type of SPD may have difficulty modulating their response to sensory input, and may be either overresponsive (hypersensitive) or underresponsive (hyposensitive) to sensory stimuli.

Hypersensitivity can lead to a variety of symptoms, such as avoiding certain textures or foods, feeling overwhelmed in crowded or noisy environments, and becoming easily agitated or distressed in response to sensory input. On the other hand, hyposensitivity can lead to symptoms such as seeking out sensory input (such as spinning or rocking), having a high pain threshold, and being unaware of changes in temperature or other sensations.

Sensory Discrimination Disorder

Sensory Discrimination Disorder is a type of SPD in which the brain has difficulty distinguishing between different types of sensory input. This can manifest as difficulty with tasks such as identifying different textures, recognizing faces or objects, and distinguishing between different sounds or tones.

Individuals with Sensory Discrimination Disorder may also have difficulty with fine motor tasks that require precise movements, such as buttoning clothes or using utensils. Additionally, they may struggle with tasks that require visual-spatial processing, such as reading maps or navigating unfamiliar environments.

Sensory-Based Motor Disorder

Sensory-Based Motor Disorder is a type of SPD in which the brain has difficulty using sensory input to guide motor movements. This can manifest as difficulty with tasks such as riding a bike, climbing stairs, or participating in sports activities. Individuals with this type of SPD may also have difficulty with balance, coordination, and overall motor planning.

Symptoms of Sensory-Based Motor Disorder may also include difficulty with tasks such as handwriting, cutting with scissors, and buttoning clothes. Additionally, individuals with this type of SPD may struggle with tasks that require both fine and gross motor coordination, such as playing a musical instrument or engaging in complex art projects.

Diagnosis and Treatment

Diagnosing SPD can be challenging, as it is often mistaken for other conditions such as autism spectrum disorder or attention deficit hyperactivity disorder (ADHD). However, a qualified healthcare provider, such as an occupational therapist, can conduct a comprehensive evaluation to assess sensory processing abilities and identify specific symptoms and signs of SPD.

Treatment for SPD typically involves a multidisciplinary approach that may include occupational therapy, speech therapy, and behavioural therapy. Sensory integration therapy, which involves engaging in sensory-rich activities to help individuals learn to process and regulate sensory input, is often used to address the symptoms of SPD.

Additionally, individuals with SPD may benefit from a variety of sensory tools and accommodations to create a sensory-friendly environment, such as weighted blankets or compression clothing, noise-cancelling headphones, and designated quiet spaces for sensory breaks.

In conclusion, Sensory Processing Disorder is a complex condition that can impact individuals in a variety of ways. Understanding the different types of SPD and their corresponding symptoms and signs is important in order to receive an accurate diagnosis and identify effective treatment options. With the right resources and support, individuals with SPD can learn to manage their symptoms and thrive in a sensory-rich world.

Sensory Integration Assessment and Diagnosis

Sensory Integration (SI) assessment and diagnosis is an important step in identifying and treating Sensory Processing Disorder (SPD). It involves a comprehensive evaluation of an individual's sensory processing abilities, including their strengths and weaknesses, to determine the specific type and severity of SPD.

Assessment Process

The assessment process typically begins with a comprehensive intake interview, during which the clinician gathers information about the individual's medical history, developmental milestones, and current sensory processing challenges. This information is used to guide the assessment process and to develop a customized treatment plan.

The SI assessment itself typically involves a combination of standardized tests, observations, and parent and caregiver input. The specific assessments used may vary depending on the individual's age, developmental level, and sensory processing challenges.

Standardized tests may include the Sensory Integration and Praxis Tests (SIPT), which evaluates a range of sensory processing abilities, including tactile, proprioceptive, and vestibular processing. The Test of Sensory Functions in Infants (TSFI) Is another commonly used assessment tool for infants and young children.

Observations of the individual in various environments and during different activities can provide valuable information about their sensory processing challenges and strengths. This may involve observing the individual during play, self-care activities, and academic tasks.

Parent and caregiver input is also an important component of the assessment process. This may involve completing questionnaires and providing detailed information about the individual's sensory processing challenges in various environments and situations.

Diagnosis

Once the assessment is complete, the clinician will use the information gathered to make a diagnosis of SPD. The diagnosis will be based on the specific type and severity of SPD identified during the assessment, as well as the individual's unique sensory processing profile.

There are three main types of SPD, as previously discussed: Sensory Modulation Disorder, Sensory Discrimination Disorder, and Sensory-Based Motor Disorder. The specific type of SPD diagnosed will depend on the individual's specific symptoms and challenges.

In addition to identifying the type of SPD, the clinician will also determine the severity of the condition. Severity can range from mild to severe and can impact an individual's daily functioning in various ways.

Treatment

Once a diagnosis has been made, a customized treatment plan will be developed to address the individual's specific sensory processing challenges. Treatment may involve a variety of interventions, including occupational therapy, speech therapy, and behavioural therapy.

Sensory integration therapy is often used to address SPD symptoms. This may involve engaging in sensory-rich activities designed to help the individual learn to process and regulate sensory input. Sensory integration therapy can be tailored to address specific sensory challenges, such as difficulty with tactile or vestibular processing.

In addition to therapy, individuals with SPD may benefit from sensory tools and accommodations to create a sensory-friendly environment. These may include weighted blankets or vests, compression clothing, noise-cancelling headphones, and designated quiet spaces for sensory breaks.

Conclusion

Sensory integration assessment and diagnosis is a critical step in identifying and treating Sensory Processing Disorder. A comprehensive assessment can provide valuable information about an individual's specific sensory processing challenges and strengths, which can guide the development of a customized treatment plan. With the right interventions and support, individuals with SPD can learn to manage their symptoms and thrive in a sensory-rich world.

Causes of Sensory Processing Disorder

Sensory Processing Disorder (SPD) is a complex neurological condition that affects how an individual processes sensory information. The exact cause of SPD is not fully understood, but there are several theories that may contribute to the development of the disorder.

Genetic Factors

Research suggests that genetic factors may play a role in the development of SPD. Studies have found that SPD tends to run in families, indicating that there may be a genetic component to the disorder. It is thought that certain genes may contribute to the way an individual's brain processes sensory information.

Brain Development

SPD is believed to result from atypical development of the brain's sensory processing systems. During normal brain development, sensory experiences help to shape the neural connections in the brain that are responsible for processing sensory information. In individuals with SPD, there may be disruptions or delays in the development of these neural connections.

Environmental Factors

Environmental factors may also contribute to the development of SPD. Exposure to toxins, such as lead or mercury, during critical periods of brain development may interfere with the development of the brain's sensory processing systems. Prenatal exposure to alcohol or drugs may also increase the risk of SPD.

Prematurity and Low Birth Weight

Premature birth and low birth weight have been identified as risk factors for SPD. Infants who are born prematurely or with a low birth weight may be more susceptible to disruptions in brain development, including the development of the sensory processing systems.

Medical Conditions

Certain medical conditions have been linked to the development of SPD. For example, children with autism spectrum disorder (ASD) are more likely to also have SPD. Other medical conditions that have been associated with SPD include attention deficit hyperactivity disorder (ADHD), developmental coordination disorder (DCD), and anxiety disorders.

Trauma

Trauma has also been identified as a potential contributor to the development of SPD. Physical or emotional trauma during critical periods of brain development may interfere with the development of the brain's sensory processing systems. For example, children who have experienced abuse or neglect may be more likely to develop SPD.

Nutritional Factors

Nutritional factors may also contribute to the development of SPD. Research has suggested that deficiencies in certain nutrients, such as zinc or vitamin D, may impact the development of the brain's sensory processing systems.

Conclusion

Sensory Processing Disorder is a complex neurological condition that affects how an individual processes sensory information. While the exact cause of SPD is not fully understood, there are several theories that may contribute to the development of the disorder, including genetic factors, disruptions in brain development, environmental factors, prematurity and low birth weight, medical conditions, trauma, and nutritional factors.

Understanding the potential causes of SPD is an important step in developing effective interventions and treatment strategies for individuals with this condition. If you suspect that you or a loved one may have SPD, it is important to seek evaluation and treatment from a qualified healthcare provider.

The Importance of Early Intervention

Early intervention is critical for children with sensory processing disorder (SPD). The sooner SPD is identified and treated, the better the chances for a positive outcome. Early intervention can help children with SPD develop better sensory integration skills, improve their ability to function in daily activities, and prevent the development of secondary problems, such as anxiety, depression, or behaviour problems.

Identifying SPD Early

The first step in early intervention is identifying SPD as early as possible. This can be challenging, as the symptoms of SPD can vary widely between individuals and may be mistaken for other conditions. However, there are certain red flags that parents and healthcare providers should watch for, including:

Over or underreacting to sensory stimuli

Difficulty with coordination and balance

Fear or avoidance of certain sensory experiences

Difficulty with social interactions or communication

Behavioural issues or emotional regulation problems

If parents or healthcare providers suspect that a child may have SPD, they should seek evaluation and diagnosis from a qualified healthcare professional, such as an occupational therapist or developmental pediatrician.

Benefits of Early Intervention

Early intervention for SPD can provide numerous benefits for children and their families. Some of the key benefits include:

Improved Sensory Integration Skills: Early intervention can help children develop better sensory integration skills, allowing them to better process and respond to sensory stimuli. This can lead to improvements in coordination, balance, motor skills, and overall functional abilities.

Improved Quality of Life: By addressing SPD early, children can learn to cope with sensory stimuli and participate more fully in daily activities. This can lead to improved self-esteem, confidence, and overall quality of life.

Prevention of Secondary Problems: Children with untreated SPD may be at risk for developing secondary problems, such as anxiety, depression, or behaviour problems. Early intervention can help prevent the development of these problems by addressing the underlying sensory processing issues.

Improved Social and Communication Skills: Children with SPD may have difficulty with social interactions or communication. Early intervention can help improve these skills by addressing the underlying sensory processing issues.

Support for Families: Early intervention can also provide support for families, who may be struggling to understand and cope with their child's sensory processing challenges. By addressing SPD early, families can access resources and support to help them better understand and manage their child's condition.

Types of Early Intervention

There are several types of early intervention that may be used for children with SPD, depending on their individual needs and challenges. Some common types of early intervention for SPD include:

Sensory Integration Therapy: Sensory integration therapy is a type of occupational therapy that uses sensory experiences to help children with SPD develop better sensory processing skills. The therapy may include activities such as swinging, jumping, and playing with sensory materials.

Parent Education: Educating parents about SPD and how to support their child's sensory processing needs can be an important part of early intervention. This may include strategies for managing sensory overload, creating a sensory-friendly home environment, and promoting sensory play and exploration.

Behavioural Therapy: Behavioural therapy may be used to address behavioural issues that are related to SPD, such as anxiety, aggression, or emotional dysregulation. This may include cognitive-behavioural therapy or other forms of psychotherapy.

Medication: In some cases, medication may be used to help manage the symptoms of SPD, particularly if the child has comorbid conditions such as ADHD or anxiety.

Conclusion

Early intervention is critical for children with sensory processing disorder. By identifying SPD early and providing appropriate intervention, children can develop better sensory integration skills, improve their functional abilities, and prevent the development of secondary problems. There are several types of early intervention that may be used for children with SPD, depending on their individual needs and challenges. If you suspect that your child may have SPD, it is important to seek evaluation and treatment from a qualified healthcare professional.

The Impact of Sensory Processing Disorder on Learning

Sensory processing disorder (SPD) can have a significant impact on a child's ability to learn and succeed in school. Children with SPD may struggle with attention, focus, and organization, which can make it difficult to keep up with their peers academically. Additionally, the sensory challenges associated with SPD can make it difficult for children to engage with classroom materials and participate in learning activities.

Attention and Focus Challenges

Children with SPD may have difficulty filtering out irrelevant sensory stimuli and focusing on the task at hand. This can make it challenging for them to pay attention in class and stay focused on academic tasks. Children with SPD may also be more easily distracted by sensory stimuli in their environment, such as noise or movement, which can interfere with their ability to learn and retain information.

Organization and Planning Challenges

SPD can also impact a child's ability to organize and plan their work. Children with SPD may struggle with task initiation and completion, time management, and prioritization. They may also have difficulty with executive functioning skills, such as working memory and cognitive flexibility, which can make it difficult to adapt to new learning situations and concepts.

Participation and Engagement Challenges

The sensory challenges associated with SPD can make it difficult for children to participate in classroom activities and engage with academic materials. For example, a child with tactile sensitivity may struggle to participate in a hands-on science experiment, while a child with auditory sensitivity may find it difficult to concentrate during a lecture. Additionally, children with SPD may have difficulty with social interactions, which can impact their ability to work collaboratively with peers and engage in group learning activities.

Strategies for Supporting Learning

While SPD can present significant challenges to learning, there are strategies that can be used to support children with SPD in the classroom. Some of these strategies include:

Sensory Modifications: Sensory modifications can be made to the classroom environment to reduce sensory overload and help children with SPD engage more fully in learning activities. This may include using earplugs or headphones to block out noise, providing fidget toys or stress balls for children who need to move their hands, or using textured materials to help children with tactile sensitivities engage with academic materials.

Visual Supports: Visual supports, such as visual schedules, checklists, and graphic organizers, can help children with SPD stay organized and focused on academic tasks. Visual supports can also be used to help children understand classroom expectations and follow classroom routines.

Accommodations and Modifications: Accommodations and modifications, such as extended time on tests, preferential seating, or alternative assessments, can help children with SPD succeed academically. It is important to work with the child's teacher and school to identify and implement appropriate accommodations and modifications.

Social Skills Instruction: Social skills instruction can help children with SPD develop the social skills they need to work collaboratively with peers and participate in group learning activities. Social skills instruction may include role-playing, social stories, and other strategies for teaching social skills in a structured, supportive environment.

Conclusion

Sensory processing disorder can have a significant impact on a child's ability to learn and succeed in school. Children with SPD may struggle with attention, focus, organization, and engagement, which can make it challenging to keep up with their peers academically. However, with appropriate accommodations, modifications, and supports, children with SPD can succeed academically and reach their full potential. It is important for parents, educators, and healthcare professionals to work together to identify and implement strategies for supporting children with SPD in the classroom.

Sensory Processing Disorder and Behaviour

Sensory processing disorder (SPD) can manifest in a variety of behavioural symptoms that can be challenging for parents, caregivers, and educators to manage. Children with SPD may exhibit behaviours such as sensory seeking, sensory avoidance, or sensory overload, which can impact their ability to participate in daily activities and engage in social interactions.

Sensory Seeking Behaviours

Sensory seeking behaviours are characterized by a desire for increased sensory input. Children with SPD may engage in sensory seeking behaviours in order to regulate their sensory system and achieve a more optimal level of arousal. Examples of sensory seeking behaviours include:

Tactile seeking behaviours, such as touching or rubbing objects or other people

Proprioceptive seeking behaviours, such as jumping or crashing into objects

Vestibular seeking behaviours, such as spinning or rocking

While sensory seeking behaviours can be beneficial in helping children regulate their sensory system, they can also be disruptive and challenging for parents and caregivers to manage. It is important for parents and caregivers to provide appropriate sensory input and opportunities for sensory exploration in order to help children regulate their sensory system in a positive way.

Sensory Avoidance Behaviours

Sensory avoidance behaviours are characterized by a desire to avoid or withdraw from certain sensory stimuli. Children with SPD may engage in sensory avoidance behaviours in order to avoid sensory overload or discomfort. Examples of sensory avoidance behaviours include:

Tactile avoidance behaviours, such as avoiding certain textures or clothing

Auditory avoidance behaviours, such as covering ears or avoiding loud noises

Visual avoidance behaviours, such as avoiding bright or flashing lights

While sensory avoidance behaviours may provide temporary relief from sensory discomfort, they can also limit a child's ability to engage in daily activities and participate in social interactions. It is important for parents and caregivers to work with the child to identify and understand the sensory stimuli that are challenging for them and to provide appropriate accommodations and modifications in order to support their participation in daily activities.

Sensory Overload Behaviours

Sensory overload behaviours are characterized by a state of sensory overload or overwhelm. Children with SPD may experience sensory overload when they are exposed to too much sensory input or when they are unable to regulate their sensory system. Examples of sensory overload behaviours include:

Meltdowns or tantrums

Aggression or irritability

Shutdown or withdrawal

Sensory overload behaviours can be challenging for parents and caregivers to manage and can impact the child's ability to participate in daily activities and engage in social interactions. It is important for parents and caregivers to work with the child to identify and understand their triggers for sensory overload and to provide appropriate accommodations and strategies for managing sensory overload when it occurs.

Strategies for Managing Sensory Processing Disorder Behaviours

There are a variety of strategies that can be used to manage sensory processing disorder behaviours. Some of these strategies include:

Sensory accommodations: Providing appropriate sensory input and opportunities for sensory exploration can help children regulate their sensory system in a positive way. Sensory accommodations may include using weighted blankets or vests, providing fidget toys or stress balls, or using sensory rooms or quiet spaces.

Visual supports: Visual supports, such as visual schedules, checklists, and social stories, can help children understand expectations and routines and provide a sense of predictability and structure.

Social skills instruction: Social skills instruction can help children develop the social skills they need to participate in social interactions and engage in group activities. Social skills instruction may include role-playing, social stories, and other strategies for teaching social skills in a structured, supportive environment.

Positive behaviour support: Positive behaviour support focuses on reinforcing positive behaviours and teaching replacement behaviours for challenging behaviours. Positive behaviour support may include using rewards or incentives for positive behaviours, teaching self-regulation strategies, or providing clear and consistent consequences for challenging behaviours.

Sensory Processing Disorder and Social Interaction

Sensory processing disorder (SPD) can impact a child's ability to engage in social interactions and form positive relationships with peers and adults. Children with SPD may experience challenges with social communication, social skills, and social awareness, which can make it difficult for them to participate in group activities and navigate social situations.

Social Communication and Sensory Processing Disorder

Social communication refers to the ability to use language and nonverbal cues to communicate with others. Children with SPD may experience challenges with social communication, including difficulty understanding social cues and body language, and difficulty using appropriate language and tone in social situations. These challenges can make it difficult for children to form positive relationships with peers and adults and may result in feelings of isolation and frustration.

Sensory Processing Disorder and Social Skills

Social skills refer to the ability to interact with others in a positive and meaningful way. Children with SPD may experience challenges with social skills, including difficulty initiating conversations, sharing and taking turns, and understanding the perspective of others. These challenges can make it difficult for children to participate in group activities and may result in social isolation and difficulty forming positive relationships.

Sensory Processing Disorder and Social Awareness

Social awareness refers to the ability to understand and interpret social situations and cues. Children with SPD may experience challenges with social awareness, including difficulty understanding social norms and expectations, and difficulty recognizing the emotions and feelings of others. These challenges can make it difficult for children to navigate social situations and may result in social isolation and difficulty forming positive relationships.

Strategies for Supporting Social Interaction in Children with SPD

There are a variety of strategies that can be used to support social interaction in children with SPD. Some of these strategies include:

Sensory accommodations: Providing appropriate sensory input and opportunities for sensory exploration can help children regulate their sensory system and reduce sensory overload, which can improve their ability to engage in social interactions.

Social skills instruction: Social skills instruction can help children develop the social skills they need to participate in social interactions and engage in group activities. Social skills instruction may include role-playing, social stories, and other strategies for teaching social skills in a structured, supportive environment.

Peer mentoring: Peer mentoring programs can provide children with opportunities to form positive relationships with peers who can provide support and guidance in social situations.

Family education and support: Providing education and support to families can help them understand their child's challenges with social interaction and provide them with strategies for supporting their child's social development.

Occupational therapy: Occupational therapy can provide children with sensory processing challenges with individualized support and strategies for improving their social skills and social interaction.

Conclusion

Sensory processing disorder can impact a child's ability to engage in social interaction and form positive relationships with peers and adults. Understanding the challenges associated with social communication, social skills, and social awareness can help parents, caregivers, and educators provide appropriate support and strategies for promoting social interaction and positive social development in children with SPD. By providing appropriate sensory accommodations, social skills instruction, peer mentoring, family education and support, and occupational therapy, children with SPD can develop the skills they need to participate in social interactions and form positive relationships.

Sensory Processing Disorder and Anxiety

Sensory processing disorder (SPD) can often be accompanied by anxiety, particularly in children. SPD can cause children to become easily overwhelmed by sensory stimuli, leading to feelings of anxiety and even panic. Additionally, the challenges associated with SPD, such as difficulty with social interactions, can also contribute to anxiety in children.

Symptoms of Anxiety in Children with SPD

Children with SPD who experience anxiety may exhibit a variety of symptoms, including:

Excessive worry or fear

Difficulty sleeping or nightmares

Avoidance of certain activities or places

Difficulty concentrating or staying focused

Physical symptoms such as stomachaches or headaches

Difficulty with transitions or changes in routine

It is important to note that anxiety can manifest differently in different children, and not all children with SPD will experience anxiety.

Causes of Anxiety in Children with SPD

There are several factors that can contribute to anxiety in children with SPD, including:

Sensory overload: Children with SPD can become easily overwhelmed by sensory stimuli, such as loud noises, bright lights, or strong smells. This can lead to feelings of anxiety and panic.

Difficulty with social interactions: Children with SPD may struggle with social interactions, leading to feelings of isolation and anxiety.

Lack of control: Children with SPD may feel that they have little control over their environment or their sensory experiences, which can lead to feelings of anxiety.

Previous negative experiences: Children with SPD may have had negative experiences in the past, such as being overwhelmed by sensory stimuli or experiencing social rejection, which can contribute to anxiety.

Strategies for Managing Anxiety in Children with SPD

There are several strategies that can be used to help children with SPD manage their anxiety, including:

Sensory accommodations: Providing appropriate sensory accommodations, such as a quiet space to retreat to when feeling overwhelmed, can help children regulate their sensory system and reduce anxiety.

Cognitive-behavioural therapy: Cognitive-behavioural therapy (CBT) can help children with SPD develop strategies for managing their anxiety, such as learning to recognize and challenge negative thoughts and beliefs.

Relaxation techniques: Relaxation techniques such as deep breathing, visualization, or mindfulness can help children with SPD calm their nervous system and reduce anxiety.

Exposure therapy: Exposure therapy can help children gradually become desensitized to the sensory stimuli that trigger anxiety, reducing the intensity of their anxiety over time.

Social skills training: Social skills training can help children with SPD develop the skills they need to participate in social interactions and reduce feelings of isolation and anxiety.

Conclusion

Sensory processing disorder can often be accompanied by anxiety, particularly in children. Understanding the causes and symptoms of anxiety in children with SPD can help parents, caregivers, and educators provide appropriate support and strategies for managing anxiety. Sensory accommodations, cognitive-behavioural therapy, relaxation techniques, exposure therapy, and social skills training are all strategies that can be used to help children with SPD manage their anxiety and develop the skills they need to participate in social interactions and lead fulfilling lives. With appropriate support and intervention, children with SPD can learn to manage their anxiety and thrive.

Sensory Processing Disorder and ADHD

Sensory processing disorder (SPD) and attention deficit hyperactivity disorder (ADHD) are two conditions that often coexist in children. While SPD affects the way the brain processes sensory information, ADHD affects attention, impulsivity, and hyperactivity. The overlap between these two conditions can make it difficult to diagnose and treat children with both SPD and ADHD.

Symptoms of SPD and ADHD

Children with SPD and ADHD may exhibit a variety of symptoms, including:

Difficulty focusing or paying attention

Impulsivity or hyperactivity

Sensitivity to sensory stimuli, such as loud noises, bright lights, or strong smells

Difficulty with transitions or changes in routine

Difficulty with social interactions

Restlessness or fidgeting

Difficulty sleeping

Difficulty with fine motor skills or coordination

It is important to note that not all children with SPD or ADHD will exhibit all of these symptoms, and that symptoms can manifest differently in different children.

Causes of SPD and ADHD

The exact causes of SPD and ADHD are not fully understood, but both conditions are thought to have a genetic component. Additionally, environmental factors, such as exposure to toxins or stress during pregnancy, may increase the risk of developing these conditions.

The overlap between SPD and ADHD may be due in part to shared underlying neural mechanisms. Both conditions are thought to involve dysfunction in the prefrontal cortex, which is involved in regulating attention, impulsivity, and sensory processing.

Treatment for SPD and ADHD

Treating children with both SPD and ADHD can be challenging, as the two conditions require different approaches. However, a multimodal approach that addresses both sensory processing and attention can be effective.

Sensory accommodations, such as providing a quiet space to retreat to when feeling overwhelmed, can help children with SPD regulate their sensory system and reduce symptoms. Occupational therapy can also be helpful, as it can help children with SPD develop the skills they need to process sensory information more effectively.

For children with ADHD, behavioural therapy and medication may be recommended. Behavioural therapy can help children develop strategies for managing impulsivity and hyperactivity, while medication can help improve attention and focus.

It is important to work with a healthcare provider who is experienced in treating both SPD and ADHD to develop a comprehensive treatment plan that addresses both conditions.

Conclusion

Sensory processing disorder and attention deficit hyperactivity disorder often coexist in children, making it challenging to diagnose and treat. Understanding the shared and unique symptoms of these two conditions can help parents, caregivers, and healthcare providers develop an effective treatment plan. Sensory accommodations, occupational therapy, behavioural therapy, and medication are all strategies that can be used to manage symptoms and improve quality of life for children with SPD and ADHD. With appropriate support and intervention, children with these conditions can thrive and reach their full potential.

Sensory Processing Disorder and Autism

Sensory processing disorder (SPD) and autism spectrum disorder (ASD) are two conditions that often occur together in children. SPD involves difficulty processing sensory information, while ASD involves social communication and interaction difficulties, as well as repetitive behaviours and restricted interests. The overlap between these two conditions can make it challenging to differentiate between them and can complicate diagnosis and treatment.

Symptoms of SPD and Autism

Children with SPD and autism may exhibit a range of symptoms, including:

Sensitivity to sensory stimuli, such as loud noises, bright lights, or strong smells

Difficulty with social interaction and communication

Repetitive behaviours or restricted interests

Difficulty with transitions or changes in routine

Difficulty with motor skills or coordination

Anxiety or emotional dysregulation

Not all children with SPD or autism will exhibit all of these symptoms, and symptoms can manifest differently in different children.

Causes of SPD and Autism

The exact causes of SPD and autism are not fully understood, but both conditions are thought to have a genetic component. Additionally, environmental factors, such as exposure to toxins or stress during pregnancy, may increase the risk of developing these conditions.

The overlap between SPD and autism may be due in part to shared underlying neural mechanisms. Both conditions are thought to involve dysfunction in the processing and integration of sensory information in the brain.

Treatment for SPD and Autism

Treating children with both SPD and autism can be challenging, as the two conditions require different approaches. However, a multimodal approach that addresses both sensory processing and social communication can be effective.

Sensory accommodations, such as providing a quiet space to retreat to when feeling overwhelmed, can help children with SPD regulate their sensory system and reduce symptoms. Occupational therapy can also be helpful, as it can help children with SPD develop the skills they need to process sensory information more effectively.

For children with autism, behavioural therapy and social skills training may be recommended. Behavioural therapy can help children develop strategies for managing social interactions and emotional regulation, while social skills training can help children learn the skills they need to engage in social communication effectively.

It is important to work with a healthcare provider who is experienced in treating both SPD and autism to develop a comprehensive treatment plan that addresses both conditions.

Conclusion

Sensory processing disorder and autism spectrum disorder often occur together in children, making it challenging to differentiate between them and develop effective treatment plans.

Understanding the shared and unique symptoms of these two conditions can help parents, caregivers, and healthcare providers develop a comprehensive treatment plan that addresses both sensory processing and social communication difficulties. Sensory accommodations, occupational therapy, behavioural therapy, and social skills training are all strategies that can be used to manage symptoms and improve quality of life for children with SPD and autism. With appropriate support and intervention, children with these conditions can thrive and reach their full potential.

Strategies for Managing Sensory Overload

Sensory overload is a common experience for individuals with sensory processing disorder (SPD). It occurs when the brain is unable to filter out and process sensory information effectively, leading to a feeling of overwhelm and discomfort. Sensory overload can manifest in many different ways, including anxiety, irritability, and even physical symptoms such as headaches or nausea. Fortunately, there are strategies that can help individuals with SPD manage sensory overload and reduce its impact on daily life.

Identify Triggers

The first step in managing sensory overload is to identify the specific triggers that cause it. This may involve keeping a journal or log to track when sensory overload occurs and what factors may have contributed to it. Common triggers include loud noises, bright lights, strong smells, and crowds. Once you have identified your triggers, you can work to minimize exposure to them or develop coping strategies to manage their impact.

Create a Calming Environment

Creating a calm and sensory-friendly environment can be helpful in reducing sensory overload. This may involve adjusting the lighting, reducing noise levels, or minimizing clutter in the space. It may also involve using tools such as fidget toys, weighted blankets, or noise-cancelling headphones to help regulate sensory input.

Practice Relaxation Techniques

Relaxation techniques such as deep breathing, meditation, or yoga can be helpful in managing sensory overload. These techniques can help reduce stress and anxiety, which can exacerbate sensory overload symptoms. They can also help promote a sense of calm and balance in the body.

Develop Coping Strategies

Developing coping strategies to manage sensory overload can be an effective way to reduce its impact on daily life. This may involve developing a routine for managing triggers, such as taking breaks when in noisy or crowded environments. It may also involve using grounding techniques, such as focusing on a specific object or sensation, to help regulate the senses.

Seek Support

Seeking support from family, friends, or healthcare professionals can be helpful in managing sensory overload. Support can come in many different forms, including emotional support, practical assistance, or professional guidance. Support groups or online communities can also be a valuable source of information and support.

Engage in Physical Activity

Regular physical activity can be helpful in managing sensory overload. Exercise can help regulate the nervous system and reduce stress, which can help minimize sensory overload symptoms. Activities such as yoga, swimming, or hiking can also provide a sensory-friendly environment and promote a sense of calm and balance.

Consider Therapy

Therapy can be helpful in managing sensory overload, particularly for individuals with severe or persistent symptoms. Therapy may involve cognitive-behavioural therapy, which can help individuals develop coping strategies and manage anxiety related to sensory overload. Occupational therapy may also be helpful, as it can help individuals develop the skills they need to process sensory information more effectively.

Managing sensory overload can be challenging, but with the right strategies and support, it is possible to reduce its impact on daily life. Identifying triggers, creating a calming environment, practicing relaxation techniques, developing coping strategies, seeking support, engaging in physical activity, and considering therapy are all effective strategies for managing sensory overload in individuals with sensory processing disorder.

Sensory-Friendly Environments

Creating sensory-friendly environments can be incredibly helpful for individuals with sensory processing disorder (SPD) as it can reduce the amount of sensory overload they experience. Sensory-friendly environments are designed to be calming and comfortable and can help individuals with SPD to regulate their sensory input. Here are some strategies for creating sensory-friendly environments:

Reduce Noise: One of the main sources of sensory overload is noise. Therefore, reducing noise levels can make a significant difference in creating a sensory-friendly environment. You can use soundproofing materials such as acoustic tiles, rugs, or curtains to reduce noise levels.

Adjust Lighting: Bright or flickering lights can be overwhelming for individuals with SPD. Using natural lighting or dimming artificial lights can help create a calm environment.

Choose Calming Colors: Colors can also impact a person's sensory experience. Using calming colors such as blue, green, or lavender can help create a calming environment.

Provide Sensory Toys: Providing sensory toys such as fidget spinners, stress balls, or tactile objects can help individuals with SPD to regulate their sensory input.

Offer Sensory Breaks: Sensory breaks are essential for individuals with SPD as they allow them to take a break from overwhelming sensory input. A sensory break could involve taking a few minutes to listen to calming music, do deep breathing exercises, or engage in sensory play.

Consider Textures: Individuals with SPD may struggle with certain textures, such as scratchy fabrics or certain foods. Consider using soft fabrics, and offer a range of food textures to accommodate different sensory preferences.

Provide Weighted Items: Weighted blankets, vests, or lap pads can provide deep pressure input that can be calming for individuals with SPD.

Use Aromatherapy: Aromatherapy can also be useful in creating a sensory-friendly environment. Scents such as lavender or chamomile can be calming for some individuals.

Organize Space: A cluttered or disorganized space can be overwhelming for individuals with SPD. Keeping the space organized and tidy can create a sense of calm and order.

Communicate Clearly: Finally, it's essential to communicate clearly with individuals with SPD about the environment and any changes that may occur. Providing advance notice about any changes to the environment can help reduce anxiety and sensory overload.

In conclusion, creating sensory-friendly environments can significantly impact the quality of life for individuals with SPD. By following these strategies, individuals with SPD can better regulate their sensory input and feel more comfortable in their surroundings.

Sensory Diets and Therapy

Sensory diets and therapy are a crucial part of managing sensory processing disorder (SPD). Sensory diets are designed to provide the appropriate amount of sensory input needed for an individual with SPD to function effectively. Sensory therapy involves working with an occupational therapist who specializes in sensory processing to develop a personalized sensory diet and provide specific therapy techniques. Here's what you need to know about sensory diets and therapy:

What is a Sensory Diet?

A sensory diet is a structured program designed to provide an individual with SPD with the sensory input they need to function effectively. A sensory diet typically involves a combination of sensory activities, such as deep pressure activities, vestibular activities, tactile activities, and proprioceptive activities.

Deep pressure activities involve providing deep pressure to the body, such as through the use of a weighted blanket, compression clothing, or a deep pressure massage. These activities can help to calm and regulate the nervous system.

Vestibular activities involve movement and include activities such as swinging, bouncing on a therapy ball, or spinning. These activities can help to improve balance, coordination, and spatial awareness.

Tactile activities involve providing different textures to the body, such as sand, playdough, or textured surfaces. These activities can help to desensitize the nervous system to certain textures.

Proprioceptive activities involve providing resistance to the body, such as through pushing or pulling against a wall, lifting weights, or carrying heavy objects. These activities can help to improve body awareness and motor planning.

What is Sensory Therapy?

Sensory therapy involves working with an occupational therapist who specializes in sensory processing to develop a personalized sensory diet and provide specific therapy techniques. Sensory therapy typically involves a combination of sensory integration therapy, occupational therapy, and cognitive-behavioural therapy.

Sensory integration therapy involves providing controlled sensory input to the individual with SPD through various activities. The goal is to help the individual learn to regulate their sensory input and respond appropriately to sensory stimuli.

Occupational therapy involves helping the individual with SPD to develop the skills they need to function effectively in their daily lives. This may include developing fine motor skills, improving coordination and balance, and learning strategies for managing sensory overload.

Cognitive-behavioural therapy involves working with the individual to develop coping strategies for managing anxiety, stress, and other emotional issues related to SPD.

Benefits of Sensory Diets and Therapy

Sensory diets and therapy can provide numerous benefits for individuals with SPD, including:

Improved sensory processing and regulation: Sensory diets and therapy can help individuals with SPD to better regulate their sensory input, leading to improved function and decreased sensory overload.

Improved behaviour and social skills: By reducing sensory overload and improving sensory processing, sensory diets and therapy can improve behaviour and social skills, making it easier for individuals with SPD to interact with others.

Improved academic performance: Sensory diets and therapy can help individuals with SPD to better focus and attend to academic tasks, leading to improved academic performance.

Improved emotional well-being: Sensory diets and therapy can help individuals with SPD to better manage anxiety and stress related to sensory overload, leading to improved emotional well-being.

In conclusion, sensory diets and therapy are essential components of managing sensory processing disorder. By providing the appropriate amount of sensory input and working with an occupational therapist who specializes in sensory processing, individuals with SPD can improve their sensory processing, behaviour, academic performance, and emotional well-being.

Sensory Integration Techniques for Children

Sensory integration techniques for children are essential in helping them cope with sensory processing disorder (SPD). These techniques can improve a child's overall development and quality of life by providing them with the appropriate sensory input they need to regulate their responses to sensory stimuli. Here are some effective sensory integration techniques for children:

Sensory Diet

A sensory diet is a personalized program designed to provide a child with the right amount and type of sensory input they need to function optimally. Sensory diets may include activities such as heavy work, brushing, and joint compression to help children regulate their sensory systems.

Deep Pressure

Deep pressure activities can provide children with the necessary input to help them feel calm and organized. Activities like weighted blankets, weighted vests, and compression garments can offer deep pressure to the body.

Vestibular Input

Vestibular input helps a child regulate their balance and movement. Activities like swinging, spinning, and rocking provide the child with the vestibular input they need to feel comfortable.

Proprioceptive Input

Proprioceptive input helps a child understand where their body is in space. Activities like jumping, climbing, and pushing can provide children with proprioceptive input.

Tactile Input

Tactile input helps a child regulate their sense of touch. Activities like playing with textured materials, massaging, and using a vibrating tool can provide the child with the necessary tactile input.

Visual Input

Visual input helps a child regulate their vision. Activities like playing with light-up toys, using a light box, and playing with bubbles can provide visual input.

Auditory Input

Auditory input helps a child regulate their sense of hearing. Activities like listening to music, playing with sound-making toys, and using noise-canceling headphones can provide the necessary auditory input.

Environmental Modifications

Modifying the environment can help reduce sensory overload. Modifications like using natural lighting, creating a quiet space, and using calming colors can help create a sensory-friendly environment.

Sensory-Friendly Activities

Sensory-friendly activities can help provide children with appropriate sensory input while having fun. Activities like painting, playdough, and sensory bins can provide children with sensory input while promoting play and creativity.

Sensory Integration Therapy

Sensory integration therapy is a specialized form of therapy designed to help children with sensory processing disorder. This therapy involves providing children with the appropriate sensory input they need to improve their overall sensory functioning.

In conclusion, sensory integration techniques are essential in helping children with sensory processing disorder regulate their sensory systems. These techniques can provide children with the necessary sensory input they need to function optimally, improving their overall quality of life. It is essential to work with a trained therapist or occupational therapist to determine the appropriate sensory integration techniques for your child's unique needs.

Sensory Integration Techniques for Adults

Sensory processing disorder (SPD) is a condition that affects both children and adults. While much of the literature and focus on SPD is on children, adults with SPD also experience significant challenges in their daily lives. They may struggle with sensory overload, difficulties with social interactions, anxiety, and other issues related to sensory processing. Fortunately, there are many sensory integration techniques that can help adults with SPD manage their symptoms and improve their quality of life.

Deep Pressure Therapy: Deep pressure can help regulate the nervous system and reduce anxiety. Techniques like weighted blankets, compression vests, and weighted vests can provide deep pressure and improve sensory processing.

Sensory Diets: Sensory diets are personalized programs of sensory activities that can help individuals with SPD regulate their sensory systems. Sensory diets can include activities like swinging, bouncing on a therapy ball, or using a vibrating cushion.

Sensory Integration Therapy: Sensory integration therapy involves working with an occupational therapist to engage in activities that stimulate the senses in a controlled, safe environment. This can help individuals with SPD learn to regulate their sensory systems and improve their ability to participate in daily activities.

Meditation and Mindfulness: Practicing mindfulness and meditation can help reduce anxiety and improve sensory processing. Techniques like deep breathing, visualization, and progressive muscle relaxation can be helpful for managing sensory overload.

Yoga: Yoga is a gentle, low-impact form of exercise that can be helpful for individuals with SPD. Yoga can help reduce anxiety, improve sensory processing, and promote relaxation.

Exercise: Exercise is important for overall health and well-being, but it can also be helpful for managing SPD symptoms. Exercise can help regulate the nervous system, improve mood, and reduce anxiety.

Occupational Therapy: Occupational therapy can be a valuable resource for adults with SPD. An occupational therapist can work with individuals to develop strategies for managing sensory overload, improving sensory processing, and participating in daily activities.

Visual Schedules: Visual schedules can be helpful for individuals with SPD who struggle with transitions and changes in routine. Using a visual schedule can help individuals anticipate changes and reduce anxiety.

Sensory-Friendly Environments: Creating a sensory-friendly environment can be helpful for adults with SPD. This can include minimizing sensory distractions, using calming lighting, and reducing noise levels.

Sensory Integration Products: There are many products available that can help individuals with SPD manage their symptoms. These can include fidget toys, chewelry, noise-cancelling headphones, and other products that can provide sensory input in a controlled way.

In summary, there are many sensory integration techniques that can be helpful for adults with SPD. These techniques can help individuals manage their symptoms, improve their quality of life, and participate in daily activities with greater ease. It is important to work with a healthcare professional or occupational therapist to develop a personalized plan that meets individual needs and preferences.

Occupational Therapy for Sensory Processing Disorder

Occupational Therapy (OT) is a crucial component of the treatment plan for individuals with Sensory Processing Disorder (SPD). OT for SPD focuses on addressing the sensory processing deficits, enhancing the ability to participate in daily activities, and improving overall quality of life. This chapter discusses the role of occupational therapy in managing SPD and the various interventions used by occupational therapists.

The Role of Occupational Therapy in SPD

Occupational therapists play a critical role in the assessment and treatment of SPD. They use a range of strategies to help individuals with SPD engage in meaningful activities and develop skills necessary to participate fully in daily life. The ultimate goal of OT for SPD is to help individuals with sensory processing deficits achieve their full potential and lead fulfilling lives.

The occupational therapist assesses the individual's sensory processing abilities and determines the most effective ways to support their sensory needs. The assessment involves evaluating the individual's sensory modulation, discrimination, and integration skills. Based on the assessment results, the occupational therapist develops an individualized treatment plan.

Interventions Used by Occupational Therapists

The occupational therapist uses a range of interventions to help individuals with SPD. These interventions are tailored to the individual's unique needs and may involve a combination of sensory-based strategies, environmental modifications, and adaptive equipment.

Sensory-Based Strategies

Sensory-based strategies aim to help individuals with SPD regulate their responses to sensory input. The occupational therapist works with the individual to develop skills for processing and responding to sensory input in a more adaptive and functional manner. Sensory-based strategies may include:

Sensory integration therapy: This intervention involves providing controlled sensory input to the individual in a structured environment to help them regulate their sensory responses.

Sensory diet: A sensory diet involves a structured routine of sensory activities throughout the day to help regulate the individual's sensory system.

Therapeutic listening: This intervention involves listening to music with specific frequencies to improve the individual's ability to process sensory information.

Brushing and joint compression: This intervention involves brushing the individual's skin and applying pressure to their joints to improve sensory processing.

Environmental Modifications

Environmental modifications aim to create a sensory-friendly environment that supports the individual's sensory needs. The occupational therapist works with the individual and their family to identify environmental factors that trigger sensory overload and develop strategies to modify the environment. Environmental modifications may include:

Sensory-friendly spaces: Creating sensory-friendly spaces in the home, school, or workplace can help individuals with SPD feel more comfortable and less overwhelmed.

Visual supports: Providing visual supports such as schedules, checklists, and social stories can help individuals with SPD understand expectations and reduce anxiety.

Noise-reducing headphones: Using noise-reducing headphones can help individuals with SPD block out auditory input that may be overwhelming.

Adaptive Equipment

Adaptive equipment can help individuals with SPD participate in daily activities more easily. The occupational therapist works with the individual to identify equipment that may be helpful and provides training on how to use it. Adaptive equipment may include:

Weighted vests or blankets: These provide deep pressure input to the body, which can help regulate the individual's sensory system.

Fidget toys: Fidget toys can help individuals with SPD focus and reduce anxiety.

Adaptive utensils: These utensils have specialized handles or designs that make them easier to grip and use for individuals with motor coordination difficulties.

Conclusion

Occupational therapy is a critical component of the treatment plan for individuals with SPD. The occupational therapist uses a range of sensory-based strategies, environmental modifications, and adaptive equipment to help individuals with SPD regulate their sensory system, participate in daily activities, and achieve their full potential. With the right interventions and support, individuals with SPD can improve their sensory processing abilities and lead fulfilling lives.

Speech Therapy for Sensory Processing Disorder

Speech therapy can be an effective treatment for individuals with sensory processing disorder (SPD). Speech therapists, also known as speech-language pathologists, are trained professionals who work with individuals to improve their communication skills. In the case of individuals with SPD, speech therapy can help them overcome challenges with speech, language, and social communication.

Speech therapy can be particularly helpful for individuals with SPD who struggle with language development. This can include difficulties with receptive language (understanding language), expressive language (using language), and pragmatics (social communication skills). Speech therapists can work with individuals to improve their language skills through a variety of techniques and activities.

One common approach used in speech therapy for SPD is the use of sensory-based interventions. These interventions are designed to help individuals with SPD process sensory information more effectively, which can in turn improve their ability to communicate. For example, a speech therapist may use activities that involve touch, movement, or sound to help an individual with SPD improve their ability to process and respond to sensory information.

Another approach used in speech therapy for SPD is the use of social stories. Social stories are designed to help individuals with SPD understand and navigate social situations. They can be particularly helpful for individuals who struggle with pragmatics, or social communication skills. Social stories can be written or illustrated, and can help individuals understand social expectations and norms, as well as how to respond appropriately in social situations.

Speech therapy can also be used to address feeding and swallowing difficulties, which are common among individuals with SPD. Some individuals with SPD may be hypersensitive to certain textures or tastes, which can make eating and drinking challenging. Speech therapists can work with individuals to develop strategies to overcome these difficulties, such as gradually introducing new textures or flavors, or using sensory-based interventions to help individuals become more comfortable with different types of food and drink.

In addition to these approaches, speech therapy for SPD may also involve the use of assistive technology. For example, individuals with SPD who struggle with speech may benefit from the use of augmentative and alternative communication (AAC) devices, which can help them communicate more effectively.

Overall, speech therapy can be an important component of treatment for individuals with sensory processing disorder. By addressing language, communication, and social skills, speech therapy can help individuals with SPD overcome challenges and improve their overall quality of life.

Physical Therapy for Sensory Processing Disorder

Physical therapy is a type of treatment that focuses on improving the physical abilities of individuals who may have difficulties with movement or mobility. Physical therapy can be a helpful intervention for individuals with sensory processing disorder (SPD) who may also have difficulty with motor coordination, balance, and other physical abilities. In this chapter, we will explore how physical therapy can be used to improve sensory processing disorder symptoms.

Physical therapy for SPD is often focused on improving gross and fine motor skills, balance, coordination, and body awareness. Physical therapists use a variety of techniques and exercises to achieve these goals. One common technique used in physical therapy for SPD is proprioceptive neuromuscular facilitation (PNF) stretching, which can help to improve muscle strength and coordination. This technique involves stretching and contracting muscles in a specific sequence to improve their function.

Another technique used in physical therapy for SPD is sensory integration therapy, which involves exposing the individual to different sensory experiences to improve their ability to process sensory information. For example, a physical therapist may use swings or other equipment to provide a range of sensory input that can help to improve balance, coordination, and spatial awareness.

Physical therapy may also involve the use of equipment and devices to help individuals with SPD improve their physical abilities. For example, weighted vests or compression garments can provide deep pressure sensory input, which can help to improve body awareness and coordination. Specialized equipment, such as balance boards or therapy balls, can also be used to improve balance and coordination.

In addition to these techniques, physical therapists may also use traditional exercises to help individuals with SPD improve their physical abilities. For example, exercises that target specific muscle groups or movements, such as squats or lunges, can be used to improve strength, coordination, and balance.

One of the benefits of physical therapy for SPD is that it can be tailored to the individual's specific needs and abilities. Physical therapists work closely with individuals with SPD to develop treatment plans that are appropriate for their age, abilities, and sensory processing difficulties. They also work closely with other healthcare professionals, such as occupational therapists and speech therapists, to ensure that the individual receives comprehensive care.

Physical therapy can also be used in combination with other therapies to improve overall outcomes for individuals with SPD. For example, physical therapy may be used in conjunction with occupational therapy to improve fine motor skills, or with speech therapy to improve speech and language abilities.

In summary, physical therapy can be a helpful intervention for individuals with sensory processing disorder who have difficulties with motor coordination, balance, and other physical abilities. Physical therapists use a variety of techniques and exercises to improve gross and fine motor skills, balance, coordination, and body awareness. This therapy can be tailored to the individual's specific needs and abilities, and can be used in combination with other therapies to achieve the best outcomes.

Medications for Sensory Processing Disorder

Sensory Processing Disorder (SPD) is a condition that affects the way the brain processes sensory information. People with SPD may have difficulty with processing, integrating, and responding to sensory input in a typical manner. While there is no known cure for SPD, there are various treatment options available to help individuals manage the symptoms associated with this condition. One such treatment option is medication.

It is important to note that medication is not a cure for SPD, but rather a tool that can be used in combination with other therapies to help manage symptoms. The decision to use medication should always be made in consultation with a healthcare professional and should be based on the individual needs of the person with SPD.

There are several types of medications that may be used to treat SPD. These include:

Stimulants - Stimulants are medications that increase activity in the brain and are commonly used to treat attention deficit hyperactivity disorder (ADHD). These medications can also be helpful in treating SPD, as they can help improve attention and focus, and may also help reduce hyperactivity and impulsivity.

Antidepressants - Antidepressants are medications that are commonly used to treat depression and anxiety. They can also be effective in treating SPD, as they can help regulate mood and reduce anxiety.

Antipsychotics - Antipsychotics are medications that are commonly used to treat conditions such as schizophrenia and bipolar disorder. They can also be helpful in treating SPD, particularly in cases where the individual experiences significant behavioural issues or sensory-related anxiety.

Anxiolytics - Anxiolytics are medications that are commonly used to treat anxiety disorders. They can be helpful in treating SPD, particularly in cases where anxiety is a significant symptom.

Sleep aids - Sleep disturbances are common in individuals with SPD, and may be due to sensory-related issues. Sleep aids can be helpful in managing sleep disturbances and improving overall sleep quality.

It is important to note that medication should never be the first line of treatment for SPD. Rather, it should be used in combination with other therapies such as occupational therapy, speech therapy, and physical therapy. Medication should also be closely monitored by a healthcare professional to ensure that it is effective and that any potential side effects are identified and managed.

In addition, it is important to understand that medication may not be effective for all individuals with SPD. Each person's experience with SPD is unique, and what works for one person may not work for another. It is also important to understand that medication is not a replacement for other therapies, but rather a tool that can be used in combination with other therapies to help manage symptoms.

In conclusion, medication can be a useful tool in managing symptoms of SPD. However, it should always be used in combination with other therapies, and the decision to use medication should always be made in consultation with a healthcare professional. It is also important to remember that medication is not a cure for SPD, but rather a tool that can be used to help manage symptoms. With proper treatment and support, individuals with SPD can learn to manage their symptoms and lead happy, fulfilling lives.

The Role of Nutrition in Sensory Processing Disorder

Nutrition can play an important role in managing sensory processing disorder (SPD). While it is not a cure, the right diet can help to minimize symptoms and promote overall health and well-being. In this chapter, we will explore the connection between nutrition and SPD and discuss ways in which diet can be used as a tool to manage symptoms.

SPD affects the way the brain processes sensory information, and this can manifest in a range of symptoms, including hypersensitivity or hyposensitivity to certain stimuli, difficulty with motor coordination, and behavioural issues. While the underlying cause of SPD is not fully understood, research suggests that a variety of factors can contribute, including genetics, brain development, and environmental factors.

Nutrition is one environmental factor that can impact SPD symptoms. Many individuals with SPD have sensory-related feeding issues, such as selective eating or difficulty with certain textures. These feeding issues can lead to nutrient deficiencies and imbalances, which can further exacerbate SPD symptoms.

Research has shown that certain nutrients can play a role in brain function and development, and therefore may impact SPD symptoms. For example, omega-3 fatty acids have been shown to improve cognitive function and reduce symptoms of ADHD, a condition that commonly co-occurs with SPD. Foods rich in omega-3s include fatty fish such as salmon, as well as flaxseed and chia seeds.

Vitamins and minerals are also important for brain function and development. Zinc, for example, is critical for proper brain development and has been shown to improve attention and memory. Foods high in zinc include oysters, beef, and spinach. Magnesium is another important mineral that can impact brain function and has been linked to improved sleep, reduced anxiety, and improved mood. Foods high in magnesium include almonds, spinach, and avocados.

Another factor to consider when it comes to nutrition and SPD is food sensitivities. Many individuals with SPD also have food sensitivities or allergies, which can exacerbate symptoms. Common allergens include gluten, dairy, and soy. Eliminating these foods from the diet may help to reduce symptoms and improve overall health.

It is important to note, however, that there is no one-size-fits-all diet for individuals with SPD. Every individual is unique, and what works for one person may not work for another. It is important to work with a healthcare provider or registered dietitian who specializes in SPD to develop a personalized nutrition plan that meets individual needs and addresses any nutrient deficiencies or imbalances.

In addition to working with a healthcare provider, there are some general guidelines that can be followed to promote a healthy diet for individuals with SPD. These include:

Eating a variety of nutrient-dense foods. This includes plenty of fruits and vegetables, lean protein sources, and healthy fats.

Avoiding processed foods and artificial additives. These can exacerbate symptoms in some individuals.

Incorporating anti-inflammatory foods into the diet. Inflammation has been linked to a variety of neurological conditions, including SPD. Foods that have anti-inflammatory properties include fatty fish, leafy greens, and berries.

Staying hydrated. Dehydration can exacerbate SPD symptoms, so it is important to drink plenty of water throughout the day.

Avoiding caffeine and sugar. These can cause fluctuations in energy levels and mood, which can exacerbate SPD symptoms.

Overall, while nutrition is just one piece of the puzzle when it comes to managing SPD, it can be an important tool in reducing symptoms and promoting overall health and well-being. By working with a healthcare provider or registered dietitian to develop a personalized nutrition plan, individuals with SPD can optimize their diet to meet their unique needs and minimize symptoms.

Alternative and Complementary Therapies

Alternative and complementary therapies refer to unconventional approaches to treating various health conditions, including sensory processing disorder. These therapies are intended to complement traditional medical treatments and promote well-being. In this chapter, we will explore some of the alternative and complementary therapies that may be helpful for individuals with sensory processing disorder.

Acupuncture: Acupuncture is a traditional Chinese medicine technique that involves the insertion of thin needles into specific points on the body. It is believed to help balance the body's energy, or qi, and promote healing. Some studies have suggested that acupuncture may be helpful for individuals with sensory processing disorder by improving sleep, reducing anxiety, and decreasing sensory sensitivities.

Massage therapy: Massage therapy involves the manipulation of soft tissues in the body, such as muscles and tendons, to promote relaxation and reduce tension. Some individuals with sensory processing disorder may benefit from massage therapy, as it can help improve body awareness and reduce sensory sensitivities.

Yoga: Yoga is a mind-body practice that involves physical postures, breathing exercises, and meditation. It has been shown to be helpful for reducing anxiety and improving body awareness in individuals with sensory processing disorder.

Mindfulness meditation: Mindfulness meditation involves paying attention to the present moment in a nonjudgmental way. It has been shown to be helpful for reducing anxiety and improving attention in individuals with sensory processing disorder.

Essential oils: Essential oils are concentrated plant extracts that are believed to have therapeutic properties. Some essential oils, such as lavender, chamomile, and bergamot, are believed to promote relaxation and reduce anxiety in individuals with sensory processing disorder.

Chiropractic care: Chiropractic care involves the manipulation of the spine and other joints to promote healing and improve the functioning of the nervous system. Some individuals with sensory processing disorder may benefit from chiropractic care, as it can help improve body awareness and reduce sensory sensitivities.

Dietary supplements: Certain dietary supplements, such as omega-3 fatty acids, magnesium, and zinc, have been shown to be helpful for reducing anxiety and improving cognitive function in individuals with sensory processing disorder.

Biofeedback: Biofeedback is a technique that involves the use of sensors to monitor bodily functions, such as heart rate and breathing, and provide feedback on how to control them. It has been shown to be helpful for reducing anxiety and improving attention in individuals with sensory processing disorder.

It is important to note that while these alternative and complementary therapies may be helpful for some individuals with sensory processing disorder, they are not intended to replace traditional medical treatments. It is always important to consult with a healthcare professional before starting any new therapy or supplement regimen.

In addition, it is important to be cautious when seeking out alternative and complementary therapies. Some therapies may be ineffective, and others may be potentially harmful. It is important to do your research and work with a qualified healthcare professional to determine which therapies may be helpful and safe for you or your child.

Finally, it is important to approach alternative and complementary therapies with an open mind and a realistic expectation of their potential benefits. While some therapies may provide significant improvements, others may have limited or no effect. It is important to be patient and persistent in your efforts to find effective treatments for sensory processing disorder.

Sensory Processing Disorder in the Workplace

Sensory Processing Disorder (SPD) can be a challenging condition for adults, especially in the workplace. It can impact their ability to focus, be productive, and interact with colleagues. However, there are ways to manage SPD in the workplace to minimize its impact and help individuals with SPD succeed in their careers.

The first step in managing SPD in the workplace is to identify and understand the specific sensory challenges that the individual faces. This can include sensitivities to noise, light, touch, or certain smells. Once identified, the individual can work with their employer to make necessary adjustments to their work environment. For example, if an individual is sensitive to noise, they may request to work in a quieter area or wear noise-cancelling headphones.

Another strategy is to incorporate sensory breaks throughout the workday. These breaks can help individuals with SPD regulate their sensory system and maintain focus. Examples of sensory breaks include taking a walk outside, doing some stretching, or using a sensory tool such as a stress ball or fidget spinner.

Creating a sensory-friendly workspace is also important in managing SPD in the workplace. This can include using soft lighting, having comfortable seating, and minimizing clutter. Some individuals with SPD may also benefit from having a dedicated space for sensory input, such as a quiet room with dim lighting and comfortable seating.

Communication is key when managing SPD in the workplace. It is important for individuals with SPD to communicate their needs and challenges with their employer and colleagues. This can help to create a supportive and understanding work environment where accommodations can be made.

In addition to these strategies, there are also some legal protections for individuals with SPD in the workplace. The Americans with Disabilities Act (ADA) provides protection against discrimination based on disability, including SPD. Employers are required to provide reasonable accommodations for individuals with disabilities, including those with SPD.

Some examples of reasonable accommodations for individuals with SPD may include providing noise-cancelling headphones, allowing for a flexible work schedule, or providing a sensory-friendly workspace. It is important for individuals with SPD to communicate their needs to their employer and work together to find reasonable accommodations that work for everyone.

In conclusion, SPD can present challenges in the workplace, but there are ways to manage it and succeed in one's career. Identifying and understanding specific sensory challenges, incorporating sensory breaks, creating a sensory-friendly workspace, and communicating with employers and colleagues are all important strategies. Additionally, individuals with SPD are protected by the ADA and may be entitled to reasonable accommodations in the workplace. By working together, individuals with SPD and their employers can create a supportive and successful work environment.

Coping with Sensory Processing Disorder as a Family

Sensory Processing Disorder (SPD) is not only challenging for the individual with the condition but can also be very difficult for their families. It can impact a family's daily routines, relationships, and quality of life. Coping with SPD as a family can be challenging, but with the right tools and support, it can be managed successfully.

Communication is Key

The first step in coping with SPD as a family is open communication. It's important to discuss the challenges that come with SPD and how it impacts the family as a whole. Encourage everyone to share their feelings, frustrations, and concerns. This can help to create a supportive and understanding environment.

Education and Understanding

Educating yourself and family members about SPD is an important part of coping. Learning about the condition, its symptoms, and how it affects daily life can help family members understand what their loved one with SPD is going through. This can help to reduce frustration and misunderstandings and increase empathy and understanding.

Create a Sensory-Friendly Environment

Creating a sensory-friendly environment at home can be beneficial for everyone. This can include making small changes such as adjusting lighting, reducing clutter, and using calming colors. Providing a space where your loved one with SPD can go to relax and decompress can also be helpful.

Implement Sensory Strategies

Sensory strategies can help individuals with SPD manage their symptoms and improve their quality of life. Working with a therapist can help identify effective sensory strategies for your loved one. It's important to incorporate these strategies into daily routines and activities, so they become a natural part of daily life.

Encourage Independence

Encouraging independence is an essential part of coping with SPD as a family. Helping your loved one with SPD learn how to manage their symptoms and develop coping strategies can increase their confidence and self-esteem. It's important to allow them to take ownership of their condition and their treatment.

Seek Support

Coping with SPD can be challenging, and it's important to seek support when needed. There are many support groups and resources available for families coping with SPD. These resources can provide emotional support, advice, and guidance.

Manage Stress

Managing stress is essential for families coping with SPD. The challenges of SPD can cause stress and anxiety for both the individual with the condition and their family members. Implementing stress management techniques such as exercise, meditation, and deep breathing can help reduce stress and improve overall well-being.

Take Care of Yourself

Caring for a loved one with SPD can be emotionally and physically draining. It's important for family members to take care of themselves to avoid burnout. This can include taking time for self-care activities, seeking support from friends and family, and seeking professional help when needed.

Conclusion

Coping with SPD as a family can be challenging, but it's important to remember that there is help and support available. Communication, education, creating a sensory-friendly environment, implementing sensory strategies, encouraging independence, seeking support, managing stress, and taking care of yourself are all essential steps in coping with SPD as a family. With the right tools and support, families can successfully manage SPD and improve their quality of life.

Advocating for Children with Sensory Processing Disorder

As a parent or caregiver of a child with sensory processing disorder (SPD), it is important to be an advocate for your child's needs. Advocacy involves speaking up and fighting for your child's rights and ensuring they receive appropriate support and accommodations to meet their sensory needs.

Here are some strategies for advocating for your child with SPD:

Educate yourself: Learn as much as you can about sensory processing disorder and how it affects your child. This will help you better understand your child's needs and communicate them to others.

Communicate with your child's school: Schedule a meeting with your child's teacher, school counselor, and any other relevant staff to discuss your child's sensory needs and how they can be supported in the classroom. Provide resources and information on SPD and what works best for your child.

Request accommodations: Work with the school to develop a plan that outlines accommodations that will support your child's needs. This may include providing a sensory-friendly space for your child to take breaks, allowing your child to wear noise-cancelling headphones, or adjusting the classroom lighting.

Collaborate with healthcare providers: Work with your child's occupational therapist, speech therapist, and any other healthcare providers to develop a comprehensive plan for supporting your child's sensory needs both in and out of school.

Build a support system: Connect with other parents and caregivers of children with SPD. They can provide valuable insight and support as you navigate the challenges of advocating for your child.

Be persistent: Advocacy can be a lengthy process, but it is important to stay persistent in your efforts to ensure your child's needs are met. This may involve following up with school staff or healthcare providers, and advocating for changes if accommodations are not being implemented effectively.

Celebrate successes: Remember to celebrate the successes along the way, no matter how small. Each step forward is progress toward supporting your child's needs and improving their quality of life.

Advocating for a child with SPD can be challenging, but it is important for ensuring they receive the support and accommodations they need to thrive. By educating yourself, communicating with school staff and healthcare providers, and building a support system, you can effectively advocate for your child and improve their quality of life.

Resources for Sensory Processing Disorder

Sensory Processing Disorder (SPD) can be a challenging condition to navigate, but with the right resources, support, and education, individuals and families affected by SPD can thrive. In this chapter, we will discuss some valuable resources available to help individuals with SPD and their families.

Sensory Integration Global Network (SIGN): SIGN is an international organization that provides resources, research, and education about sensory integration and processing. They offer a directory of therapists and clinics that specialize in sensory integration and processing.

American Occupational Therapy Association (AOTA): The AOTA is a professional association for occupational therapists in the United States. They provide information and resources for individuals with SPD, including directories of certified occupational therapists who specialize in sensory integration and processing.

STAR Institute for Sensory Processing Disorder: The STAR Institute is a nonprofit organization dedicated to research, education, and treatment of sensory processing disorder. They offer a variety of resources for families and professionals, including online courses, webinars, and research studies.

Sensory Processing Disorder Foundation (SPDF): The SPDF is a nonprofit organization that provides education, research, and advocacy for individuals with SPD and their families. They offer a variety of resources, including webinars, conferences, and a sensory processing disorder checklist for parents.

SPD Parent Support: SPD Parent Support is an online community for parents of children with SPD. They offer support, resources, and a forum for parents to connect with one another and share their experiences.

Sensory Smarts: Sensory Smarts is an online resource for parents and professionals who work with children with sensory processing disorder. They offer resources and tools, including articles, checklists, and handouts.

Understanding SPD: Understanding SPD is a website and blog created by Rachel Schneider, a mother of two children with SPD. The website offers information, resources, and personal stories about living with SPD.

The Out-of-Sync Child: The Out-of-Sync Child is a book by Carol Stock Kranowitz that provides an introduction to SPD and practical strategies for managing sensory processing difficulties.

Sensational Kids: Sensational Kids is a book by Lucy Jane Miller that provides information about SPD and practical strategies for helping children with sensory processing difficulties.

Sensory Processing Disorder Resource Center: The Sensory Processing Disorder Resource Center is an online resource that provides information, resources, and a community for individuals with SPD and their families.

Sensory Processing Disorder Parent Network: The Sensory Processing Disorder Parent Network is an online community for parents of children with SPD. They offer support, resources, and a forum for parents to connect with one another and share their experiences.

Sensory Street Kids: Sensory Street Kids is an online resource that provides information and resources for parents and professionals who work with children with sensory processing difficulties.

Sensory Kids Store: The Sensory Kids Store is an online store that offers a variety of products and resources to support children with sensory processing difficulties.

Sensory Friendly Solutions: Sensory Friendly Solutions is a website that provides information and resources for individuals with SPD and their families, including sensory-friendly products, resources, and tips.

Understood: Understood is a website that provides resources and support for individuals with learning and attention issues, including SPD. They offer a variety of resources, including articles, webinars, and forums.

National Institute of Child Health and Human Development (NICHD): The NICHD is a government organization that conducts research and provides information about child development and health. They offer resources about SPD and related conditions.

National Center on Birth Defects and Developmental Disabilities (NCBDDD): The NCBDDD is a government organization that provides information and resources about developmental disabilities, including SPD.

Research and Future Directions

Sensory Processing Disorder (SPD) is a complex and often misunderstood condition that affects a significant portion of the population. While research on SPD is still in its early stages, there have been many advances in recent years that have helped us better understand the causes, symptoms, and treatments of this condition. In this chapter, we will discuss some of the most promising areas of research and future directions for the study of SPD.

Research on the Causes of Sensory Processing Disorder

One of the most significant challenges in understanding SPD has been identifying its underlying causes. Research suggests that genetics and environmental factors both play a role in the development of SPD. Studies have identified specific genes that may be associated with sensory processing difficulties, and prenatal exposure to certain substances, such as alcohol and tobacco, has been linked to an increased risk of SPD. Additionally, premature birth, low birth weight, and other factors that can affect early brain development may also contribute to the development of SPD.

Another area of research focuses on the role of the immune system in SPD. Some studies suggest that the immune system may be overactive in individuals with SPD, leading to increased inflammation and other problems. Researchers are currently investigating the relationship between the immune system, the gut microbiome, and sensory processing, which may help us better understand the mechanisms underlying this condition.

Assessment and Diagnosis of Sensory Processing Disorder

There is currently no standardized method for diagnosing SPD, which can make it difficult for individuals to access appropriate care and support. However, researchers are working to develop more reliable and valid assessment tools that can be used to identify and diagnose SPD. For example, the Sensory Processing 3-Dimensional Inventory (SP-3D) is a new tool that aims to provide a more comprehensive assessment of sensory processing difficulties by looking at how individuals respond to sensory stimuli in different contexts.

Treatments for Sensory Processing Disorder

Research on the effectiveness of treatments for SPD is ongoing, but there are several promising interventions that have been shown to be effective in improving sensory processing and reducing symptoms. One of the most commonly used interventions is sensory integration therapy, which involves working with an occupational therapist to provide individuals with sensory experiences that can help them better regulate their responses to stimuli.

Other interventions that have shown promise include cognitive-behavioural therapy, which can help individuals learn coping strategies for dealing with sensory overload, and mindfulness-based interventions, which can help individuals become more aware of their sensory experiences and develop greater control over their responses to stimuli.

Future Directions for Research

As research on SPD continues to evolve, there are several areas that researchers are focusing on to better understand this condition and develop effective treatments. Some of these areas include:

Developing a standardized diagnostic tool for SPD that can be used across different populations and settings

Identifying the specific brain regions and neural networks that are involved in sensory processing and regulation

Investigating the relationship between SPD and other conditions, such as anxiety, depression, and autism spectrum disorder

Developing more effective pharmacological interventions for individuals with SPD

Exploring the impact of sensory processing difficulties on academic and occupational outcomes, and developing strategies to support individuals with SPD in these areas.

Conclusion

While there is still much to learn about sensory processing disorder, research in recent years has helped us gain a better understanding of the causes, symptoms, and treatments of this condition. As we continue to learn more about SPD, it is likely that we will develop more effective interventions and strategies for supporting individuals with this condition. In the meantime, it is important for individuals with SPD and their families to have access to reliable information and resources that can help them better understand and cope with the challenges of living with sensory processing difficulties.

Printed in June 2023
by Rotomail Italia S.p.A., Vignate (MI) - Italy